Juliana Rockembach
Deise Soares

Paediatrics: Playful Activities in Nursing Care

Juliana Rockembach
Deise Soares

Paediatrics: Playful Activities in Nursing Care

ScienciaScripts

Imprint
Any brand names and product names mentioned in this book are subject to trademark, brand or patent protection and are trademarks or registered trademarks of their respective holders. The use of brand names, product names, common names, trade names, product descriptions etc. even without a particular marking in this work is in no way to be construed to mean that such names may be regarded as unrestricted in respect of trademark and brand protection legislation and could thus be used by anyone.

Cover image: www.ingimage.com

This book is a translation from the original published under ISBN 978-613-9-70706-5.

Publisher:
Sciencia Scripts
is a trademark of
Dodo Books Indian Ocean Ltd. and OmniScriptum S.R.L publishing group

120 High Road, East Finchley, London, N2 9ED, United Kingdom
Str. Armeneasca 28/1, office 1, Chisinau MD-2012, Republic of Moldova, Europe
Printed at: see last page
ISBN: 978-620-7-23833-0

Dedication

"To my mum, Regina, for inspiring me to love the world of children and, with all her dedication and affection, for setting me an example by aiming to make a difference in our children's lives."

Epigraph

"To all who suffer and are alone, always give a smile of joy. Don't just give them your care, but also your heart"

Mother Teresa of Calcutta

According to the Ministry of Health (1990), there are social groups that are more susceptible to health needs evidenced by morbidity and mortality records, among them the child population. It is therefore necessary to take a close look at and understand the characteristics of this target population in order to guide the planning and implementation of health actions aimed at improving the quality of care for children.

The Statute of the Child and Adolescent (ECA) defines a child as a person up to the age of twelve and adolescents as those between the ages of twelve and eighteen. Both are entitled to all the fundamental rights inherent to the human person, in order to enable their physical, mental, moral, spiritual and social development, in conditions of freedom and dignity (ECA, 2001).

Based on the ECA and the principles of the Unified Health System (SUS), the Ministry of Health aims to develop policies and techniques for comprehensive child health care. Promotion, prevention and care presuppose a commitment to providing quality of life so that children can grow and develop to their full potential.

Aiming for healthy child development and focussing on the concept of the integrality of the human being, it is necessary to understand that attention to children must be differentiated, taking into account all the characteristics involved in the process of being a child, including the act of playing. Ravelli and Motta (2005) state that it is through play that the child explores and acquires an understanding of the world in which he or she is inserted; it is through play that he or she interacts playfully with the real world. In this context, play encompasses all children's imagination, "make-believe" and play, which, according to Piaget (2010), is fundamental to the child's growth and development.

When caring for children, the importance of play must be taken into account in order to provide better quality, humanised care. According to Ravelli and Motta (2005), the essence of nursing is caring and being open to others, using theoretical scientific knowledge and sentimental expressions, relating to others with sensitivity, taking into account all their basic needs.

Playful care in nursing must have functionality in the different areas that encompass the care provided by these professionals. When it comes to hospitalisation in childhood, the importance of this activity increases. Mitre and Gomes (2004) state that hospitalisation in childhood can be a traumatic experience, as it takes children away from their daily lives and family environment and promotes a confrontation with painful procedures and limitations, leaving them with a feeling of passivity, surfacing anxieties and fears.

In this mix of feelings, health professionals are often seen by these children as someone who puts them through painful situations, assimilating them to these feelings of vulnerability and powerlessness. This highlights the importance of health education activities in this environment, which according to Queiroz and Jorge (2006), as well as treating and/or preventing illnesses, also aim to promote children's growth and development from a quality of life perspective. In the case of children, it is necessary to involve their playful universe so that knowledge can be exchanged, providing satisfactory results in the activities. As such, I base myself on Frota, et al. (2007), who state that when the nursing team approaches children in an educational way and proposes playful activities, they are seen in a different way, giving them the opportunity to experience new, non-threatening objectives.

In short, the importance of humanised, person-centred care in all its uniqueness and complexity is highlighted, emphasising the need for nurses to take playful care into account when treating children. Through the playful approach, they provide the means for the professional to be seen as someone who will do them good and for the child to understand and become active in relation to the procedures they will undergo, collaborating consciously and improving physically and emotionally.

With regard to the benefits of the research for the subjects, the study is considered to be extremely important for the child's better adaptation, acceptance and autonomy in the face of the hospitalisation process, thus reducing anguish, fear and trauma, and strengthening the relationship with the family. As well as giving continuity to healthy child development, ensuring their identity as a child, taking into account the whole universe of children's play.

I hope that this study will enable nursing students and professionals to recognise the importance and need for this sensitive and humanised approach to caring for children, contemplating the broader concept of health, providing the necessary support during hospitalisation, creating a link between the reality experienced and the imaginary world of children.

Based on the above, the following guiding question was formulated:

How do parents perceive play activities during their child's stay in paediatrics?

General Objective:

- To investigate parents' perceptions of play activities during their child's stay in paediatrics.

Specific Objectives:

- To investigate the use of playful activities by the nursing team during the child's hospitalisation;
- To identify how children experience hospitalisation through their parents' perceptions;
- To identify the benefits of using play during paediatric hospitalisation.

In this chapter, I seek theoretical support for the study. In the first section, I summarise how children develop the ability to imitate role-playing, "make-believe", as well as the ability acquired in childhood to use symbolic play and games, all of which form part of a child's universe of play. The second section focuses on the need for hospitalisation in childhood, characterising children's needs and feelings in the face of this episode and the importance of taking into account all children's needs in this scenario, including the act of playing and the presence of parents. In the third section, I look at nursing and its importance in caring for hospitalised children, emphasising the tools that nurses have at their disposal to provide care that takes into account healthy child development.

The development of play in children

"In a child's world, anything is possible: dogs and cats live together amicably and the sky can be either pink or green, depending only on the imagination" (RAVELLI ; MOTTA, 2005, p.611). This characteristic of childhood comes about through the universe of play in which children find themselves. In this context, ludic is defined as an "adjective relating to games, play, fun" (LAROUSSE ATICA, 2001. p. 613). In order to understand the child's universe of play, it is necessary to know how this formation takes place during the stages of child development.

Papalia and Olds (2006) state that there are three stages of child development. Early childhood is from birth to 2 years of age, the second childhood or pre-school period is from 3 to 6 years of age, and the third childhood or school age is from 7 to 12 years of age.

For the authors, it is from the end of early childhood and the beginning of second childhood that the child begins to develop strength and simple motor skills, such as walking alone, holding objects, talking, etc. Their behaviour is egocentric, but they understand and have a perspective on other people. They are still cognitively immature, reflecting illogical ideas about the world. Their play becomes more elaborate, their independence, self-control and self-care increase, and the family is their centre of life and other children begin to play an important role in their lives.

In early childhood, strength and motor skills improve, egocentrism decreases and they begin to think more logically and concretely. Their memory and language skills increase, and with the increase in cognitive gains, they are able to make better use of new things they are taught. Their self-image develops and begins to affect their self-esteem, and friends and family take on fundamental importance in their lives. (PAPALIA; OLDS, 2006)

In this way, Franco (2004) states that every human being has a structural organisation that gives them a characteristic of wholeness, dynamically integrating the various parts that make them up. This is also true of thought and imagination, which are made up of elements integrated into a larger structure, including the process of adapting, assimilating and accommodating ideas. According to the author, this structuring of thoughts is progressive and gradual, accompanying the stages of the child's development until adulthood, when thinking matures and the imaginary world and the real world are distinguished.

Piaget (2010) points out that the child's playful universe is formed through representative imitation and play, which includes symbolic games. Therefore, the development of the child's thinking happens along with their growth as a human being, making it possible for them to adapt and organise their structures, thus understanding who they are and what the world they are part of is like.

Development of representative imitation

For Guillaume (apud. PIAGET 2010), imitation is not a technique that comes from instinct or that is inherited from father to son: the child learns to imitate and turn this imitation into play. For Piaget (2010), learning to imitate takes place progressively during different stages of the child's development. According to the author, the first phase takes place during the first month of life and is the absence of imitation, where there is simply the reproduction of a model by simple reflex stimulated by an external stimulant. This is the case of a newborn who is stimulated by the cries of other babies in the nursery and starts crying in chorus with them. It's possible that the crying of others simply arouses an unpleasant sensation in the newborn, without them establishing a relationship between the sounds they hear and their own. In this way, it can be considered that the crying is repeated thanks to a kind of "reflex exercise" and is not imitative.

After the first month of life, the child goes through phases of maturation of the intelligence and senses. According to Rappaport (2002), during this period, the child's social interaction is very limited and imitation of an exploratory nature predominates, in which the baby seems to explore the potential of objects without the need to adapt to them. Thus, imitation takes place sporadically, requiring external stimuli, and happens simply out of a desire to continue and maintain the activity that is giving them pleasure. We can therefore perceive a primitive playful character in such attitudes, where the baby explores and continues to throw whatever causes him pleasant sensations.

After sporadic imitation, on average at 4 months of age, Piaget (2010) states that a new phase of play development begins for the baby. Imitation now takes place systematically and intentionally, where the child is able to repeat sounds and movements that are already known and visible to them. It is essentially conservative, i.e. without attempts to imitate new models, and without realising the similarity between their body and someone else's, they won't be able to imitate actions that they can't see in their own body, such as sticking out their tongue.

According to Piaget (2010), as intelligence progresses, on average between 8 and 9 months of age, babies begin to assimilate the gestures of other people to those of their own bodies, even when these gestures remain outside their field of vision, and are then able to imitate new models. However, there is still some confusion between the organs, and they can easily open and close their mouths when trying to imitate opening and closing their eyes. This confusion is resolved when the baby, for example, transforms a salivation noise into a signal that triggers the perception that the action is taking place in the mouth, translating the visual stimulus into a kinaesthetic sensation. On the basis of the above, Rappaport (2002) concludes that once children have discovered the parts of their bodies, they begin to repeat the movements, no longer in an attempt to "solve problems", but as a way of imitating and achieving pleasant sensations.

On average, from the second year of age, Piaget (2010) says that imitation proper begins, with a representative character, the child no longer needs examples, disconnecting from the current action, becoming able to imitate a series of models internally, given in the state of images or sketches of acts stored in their memory, thus reaching the beginnings of the level of representation.

From the age of 3 to 6, representational imitation expands and generalises into a spontaneous form, becomes reflexive and is integrated into the child's own intelligence. The child is able to give new meanings to people, objects or situations, depending solely on their imagination and the context in which they find themselves. According to Piaget, 2010, p. 95:

> Imitation is always an extension of intelligence, but in the sense of differentiation according to new models: the child imitates an aeroplane or a tower, etc. because they understand its meaning and are only interested in it in any relation to their own activities.

Piaget (2010, p.95) states that "with the development of social life and the exchange of thoughts, all kinds of new nuances and gradations emerge". This is how the child attaches prestige to those people who play an important role in his or her life, imitating them as such. In short, first there is the imitation of details with analyses and reconstitutions of the models and then comes the awareness of imitation, differentiating between what comes from outside and what belongs to "the self", managing to play roles, playfully interpreting reality through imitation and "make-believe".

Symbolic play

Piaget (2010) states that the evolution of play, like imitation, takes place in stages. Until the second year of life there is no symbolic play, only sensory-motor play. At this stage, the baby has not yet developed the capacity for representative imitation, and play has the function of transmitting pleasant and reflective sensations, without the character of expressing any symbolism. Papalia and Olds (2009) state that in the first few months of life, children can only deal with the parts of their world that are captured through their five senses.

As imitation matures, the child transforms it into play. According to Piaget (2010, p. 115), "play is simply functional or reproductive assimilation", meaning that play is a symbolic transposition between the real world and the imaginary world. Based on Piaget's statement, Papalia and Olds (2009) consider that from this moment on, children are able to use symbols to make representative imitations of objects, places and people. "Thought can dart back to past events, it can jump ahead to predict the future and it can linger on what might be happening somewhere in the present" (PAPALIA; OLDS, 2009, p.223).

For Piaget (2010), from the age of 3, play and imitation take on a symbolic character in the child's life, taking on a form, rules and dimension, having the capacity to represent the situations they experience and serving as a way of creating a particular and individual reality. For example, the symbolic game of "playing with dolls" is a typical case of exercising family tendencies, particularly the maternal instinct. If we analyse in more detail, we can see in this action that the girl imitates and represents the characteristics of her own mother.

> The doll only serves as an opportunity for the child to symbolically relive their own existence [...] in order to better assimilate its various aspects, to resolve everyday conflicts and to fulfil the set of desires that remain unfulfilled. Thus, we can be sure that all the happy or upsetting events that occur in the child's life will be reflected in their dolls (PIAJET, 2010, p. 140).

When it comes to playing with dolls, Rappaport (2002) also states that it is a way of offering the child not only the opportunity to bring out their maternal instincts or to learn cultural norms for performing the female role, but above all it gives the child the opportunity to better deal with the daily conflicts they experience or to fulfil their unsatisfied desires. As she plays out her role as mother, she mentally works through the anxieties, joys, etc. that she experienced with her real mother.

In addition to this example, Rappaport (2002) also gives the case of a child who has been ill, who has had to undergo medical treatment and surgical procedures and, through symbolic play, plays at being a doctor or nurse, being able to give an injection to their doll by repeating the words "it won't hurt". Thus, by repeating the situation, the child becomes stronger in terms of structuring, creating a new situation through their imaginary world, now less harsh and milder.

Thus, not only in the case of playing with dolls, but in any other symbolic play activity carried out by children, it can be understood that play is a construction of symbols and images based on the child's own life, where it acquires multiple functions, being a basic child need, providing healthy child development, being used as a form of expression and a means of giving vent to their feelings.

Childhood Hospitalisation and Play in Hospital

Hospitalisation is characterised by Frota et al. (2007) as an unpleasant time, bringing with it feelings of fragility, impotence and fear. It is a difficult experience for anyone, and one that intensifies when that person is a child, surrounded by their world of imagination and symbolism, "their mind can go beyond the here and now" (PAPALIA; OLDS, 2009, p.223). Perceiving in a particular and unique way the new experiences they will encounter during the period they will be away from home.

Mitre and Gomes (2004) state that the need to be hospitalised during childhood can be a painful experience for the child, as it takes them away from their daily life and family environment and leads to a confrontation with pain, painful procedures and physical limitations, where they are forced to passively accept the activities proposed by the healthcare team.

The need arises to adapt to new schedules and routines, to trust previously unknown people and to stay in a room where they are deprived of all the activities that characterise their life as a child. With this departure from their daily lives and their new condition as a patient, the child begins to have their own perception of the new reality, assimilating the health professionals as something negative, with procedures that make them feel pain, thus, for Motta and Enumo (2004), hospitalisation can affect the child's development, directly interfering in their quality of life.

When the experience is very stressful for the child, Sabatés (2008) states that they may show emotional reactions and regressions, which may have negative repercussions during and after their stay in hospital. The child may trigger behaviours that are related to the stressful situation they are experiencing as a result of the painful and difficult procedures they are faced with. According to Mitre and Gomes (2004), this emotional burden brings up feelings of guilt, punishment and fear of death, making the child feel obliged to submit to everything that is proposed to them, without the opportunity for argument, conforming to the rules demanded by the staff and the hospital institution. Ribeiro, Almeida and Borba (2008) consider that this situation can lead to emotional aggravation if the parents are not present and if the healthcare team that is caring for the child handles it appropriately.

For the child's adaptation to the hospital unit to be better, the presence of parents/guardians actively participating in this process is of the utmost importance, with nurses encouraging them to strengthen the family bond (GOÉS; CAVA, 2009). Family participation during hospitalisation was instituted in 1990 by law 8.069 of the ECA, due to the need and benefits for the child of full-time parent/guardian accompaniment during hospitalisation.

According to Goés and Cava (2009), the full-time presence of parents/guardians in the hospital environment, their participation in care and the relationship between children, parents and professionals have led to new ways of planning care for hospitalised children. From this perspective, the focus is broadened, and it is necessary to look from a holistic perspective in a process of producing relationships and interventions that go beyond clinical care (COLLET, 2004).

In order for the child to adapt and with comprehensive care in mind, it is necessary for them to have tools at their disposal that they are familiar with and that remind them of their day-to-day life and the characteristics of their routine. According to Frota et al. (2007), one of the ways of clarifying this current change for children is through the use of playful activities, which can help to alleviate fears and anxieties, allowing them to reveal what they feel and think to their parents and the healthcare team through play.

According to Ribeiro, Almeida and Borba (2008), play is usually a form of entertainment, of creating a world where anything is possible and everything takes on a meaning of its own. It is a basic childhood need and the means by which children develop physically, emotionally, cognitively and socially. In this way, I refer to Mitre and Gomes (2004), who characterise play as a possibility for making changes in the daily life of hospitalisation, because it is through play that children produce their own unique reality. It is through a pendulum movement between the world of reality and the world of imagination that the barriers of illness and the limits of time and space are overcome.

In this way, the act of playing emerges as a way of bringing this child's universe and the hospital environment closer together. I draw on Mitre and Gomes (2004) to say that play can be a link, creating the possibility for children to express their feelings, preferences, fears and habits; it is a mediation between the familiar world and the new situations present in their lives. Frota et al. (2007) report that the act of playing is an attempt to transform the hospital environment, minimising the psychological damage caused by negative experiences, facilitating access to symbolic, playful activity and the psychic elaboration of the daily experiences of hospitalisation.

The behaviour of playing gives these children a new opportunity to see their reality, playfully modifying their environment. For Mello and Valle (2008), playing in hospital is ideal for children to vent their feelings mobilised by hospitalisation, as well as helping with the development process. For Mitre (2000), play is also seen as an activity capable of promoting the continuity of children's development, as well as the possibility for hospitalised children to better elaborate on this specific moment in their lives.

> Sometimes, in an attempt to understand the new routine, the child plays at being a nurse and a doctor. The patients are the dolls, stuffed animals and friends in the room. With clothes, masks, hospital materials such as thermometers and stethoscopes, the child plays and represents their own condition as a hospitalised child. (KISHIMOTO, apud MELO; VALLE, 2008, p.59)

This highlights the importance of taking into account all the playfulness in which the child is involved, including in the hospital environment, which according to Frota et al. (2007) is a stressful and traumatic experience for the child, reflecting on their behaviour during and after their stay in the hospital environment.

Nursing and caring for hospitalised children

The concept of health was broadened in 1990 with the approval of Organic Health Law No. 8080 in article 196, which came to be seen as the result of various determining and conditioning factors, moving from a biologicist model centred on pathology and the biological body, to a broad model where the human being is seen in all its dimensionality and complexity (BRASIL, 2010).

With this broadening of the concept of health comes the need to approach the human being in a holistic way, taking into account their entire conceptual system, which according to Waldow, Lopes and Meyer (1995) is surrounded by individuality, uniqueness, originality and totality. With physical, intellectual, emotional, social and spiritual attributes and potential. The human being is intentional, creative, with inherent rights to achieve their own development, interests and goals.

Therefore, the nursing team must keep in mind the real meaning of the care they will be providing. Care, which according to Boff (2011) means care, solicitude, diligence, zeal, good treatment. It is a fundamental action of concern and restlessness in the sense of responsibility, knowing that the basis of nursing is care, attention to others and understanding the physical and emotional needs of those being cared for, being consistent with the new concept of health.

Therefore, when dealing with children's health, the nursing team needs to understand children's characteristics and the needs that need to be met.

> Nursing care for these children must go beyond providing physical care and the knowledge that nurses must have about their illness and the diagnostic or therapeutic interventions carried out. It must also take into account their emotional and social needs, including the use of appropriate communication and relationship techniques, among which the play situation stands out (RIBEIRO; ALMEIDA; BORBA, 2008, p.65).

For the authors mentioned above, understanding that play is a basic need becomes essential for the nursing team caring for children, where this activity must be present in the hospital environment, and should be valued as much as hygiene care, technical procedures, food and medication. Care for children must be committed not only to their illness, but based on the new concept of health, satisfying their needs as a human being who is growing and developing.

Play in nursing care is recommended and regulated by the Federal Nursing Council in Resolution 295 of 24 October 2004, Article 1 of which states that:

> It is the responsibility of paediatric nurses, as part of the multi-professional healthcare team, to use the Toy/Therapeutic Toy technique when caring for hospitalised children.

Playing in childcare is seen as something that goes beyond providing pleasurable moments. According to Ribeiro, Almeida and Borba (2008), play represents a means of relieving the tensions imposed by hospitalisation and being ill. In addition, it is a means of communication through which nurses can give explanations and guidance on the procedures that will be carried out, as well as receive information from the child about how they feel and what the situations they are experiencing mean in their lives. In this way, nurses are able to set goals and design nursing care that is specifically targeted at the child, meeting their real needs.

In order to improve the quality of care provided to children, Frota et al. (2007) state that the nursing team has tools at their disposal that can provide experiences with new objectives, feelings, sensations and non-threatening activities. Thus, play emerges as a tool capable of changing the child's perception of the health professional, who from now on is seen not just as someone who proposes and carries out painful procedures, but as someone who also provides joyful moments and who understands the universe in which the child is inserted, actively participating in their symbolic constructions, speaking in their playful language.

In addition, for the authors, the support of those who care for the child is essential for their adaptation to the hospital environment and the treatments they undergo, as the differentiated approach contributes to their adaptation to the new daily routine. The professional-play-child triad interconnects purposes and expectations, facilitating positive interaction. For Mitre and Gomes (2004), play is seen as an instrument that guarantees the child's adherence to treatment. It is a vehicle for communication between the nursing professional and the child, where the nurse will create bonds in order to provide information, show and demystify procedures through health education aimed specifically at these children.

Since 1997, health education has been characterised by Candeias as combinations of learning experiences designed to facilitate voluntary actions conducive to health, triggering changes in individual behaviour. The word combination emphasises the importance of combining multiple factors of human behaviour with learning experiences and educational interventions. The term outlined distinguishes the process of health education from any other process, presenting it as a systematically planned activity. Facilitate means to predispose, enable and reinforce. Voluntary action means without coercion and with full understanding and acceptance of the educational objectives, adopting behavioural measures to achieve an intentional effect on one's own health.

In order to achieve the goals set and the aims of educational practice in health, it is essential to propose educational actions that are sensitive to the emerging needs of the subjects. Goés and Cava (2009) state that the pedagogical methodology to be adopted must take as its starting point systematic knowledge of the reality in which the subjects are inserted. They are invited to leave their silence and share their life experiences, stressing that dialogue is an essential and necessary condition for educational practice to take place.

This new approach to pedagogical methods is conceptualised by Freire (2006) as the Pedagogy of Problematisation, which breaks with non-reflective models of educating, based on receiving information and reproducing techniques, but instead affirms that the student learns from the reality they experience while preparing to change it.

To this end, the educator who aspires to work from this progressive perspective needs to understand that teaching is not about passing on knowledge, but about providing ways for the learner to have the ability to produce it according to their perspective (FREIRE, 2011). With this in mind, Ferraz et al. (2005) suggest the use of education as a form of care in nursing, transcending the basic precepts of care, because through education nurses enhance their ability to care. In this way, nurses can intervene constructively in the relationships developed between the subjects, educator and student, from a perspective where one learns from the other.

When it comes to children's health, Queroz and Jorge (2006) define health education as not only treating and/or preventing illnesses, but also promoting children's growth and development from a quality of life perspective. Goés and Cava (2009) state that in childcare there are always spaces for health education, whether it's expressing feelings, preparing for procedures, providing information about the care to be given, permeating all childcare practices and seeking to involve the family and the child's entire playful universe in this process.

As mentioned, the pedagogy of problematisation aims to break away from a model that does not take into account the full dimensionality of the human being. With this in mind, when aiming for health education where the students are hospitalised children, it is of the utmost importance to take into account their fragility, fears and anxieties pertinent to the moment in which they live. It is also necessary to realise that although they are in a different environment to their usual one, they are still children and have all the characteristics involved in this process, including their unique universe of play (FREIRE, 2006).

Thus, in caring for hospitalised children, I refer to Ribeiro, Almeida and Borba (2008) when they state that nurses should anticipate, provide and facilitate their participation in different types of play, as well as taking part in this activity, interacting educationally, taking into account the whole reality and integrality of this child, thus coherent with the concept of problematisation pedagogy.

The nurse's participation is of the utmost importance so that the child doesn't only relate to unpleasant and painful procedures, demystifying the negative image of the healthcare team, bringing better acceptance and understanding of the treatment, awakening positive feelings in the child about hospitalisation and its necessity for improving health. All this participation by nurses in the hospitalisation process and playfulness helps to establish bonds and a relationship of trust and friendship between the child being cared for and the nurse.

Research characterisation

This is a qualitative, descriptive and exploratory study. Creswell (2010) defines qualitative research as a way of exploring and understanding the meaning that individuals attribute to the problems they experience. Still on the subject of qualitative research, Leopardi (2002) states that with this type of study it is possible to understand a situation from the perspective of the subjects, so it is pertinent to use this method when the intention is to know the meaning of a variable and not to count it.

Minayo (2010) defines a study as descriptive when it is carried out completely freely and describes all the characteristics of a population or phenomenon.

According to Minayo (2010), a study is exploratory when it clarifies and modifies concepts and ideas with the intention of getting involved in the study by choosing, constructing and investigating the topic.

Research location

This study was carried out in a paediatric inpatient unit at a university hospital in a city in the south of Rio Grande do Sul.

The hospital only meets SUS demand and has an adult ICU (Intensive Care Unit), paediatric and neonatal ICU, PIDI (Interdisciplinary Home Internment Programme), clinical, surgical and paediatric internment units.

The paediatric unit has five wards, one of which is for isolation, one for semi-intensive care, one for newborns, one for respiratory disorders and the last one, which covers infants to older children. The patients admitted to the study unit are full-term and premature newborns, infants, pre-schoolers, schoolchildren and pre-adolescents up to the age of eleven.

The nursing team on the morning and afternoon shifts consists of one nurse and six nursing technicians. On the night shift there are three nurses and fifteen technicians, divided into three teams. There are also nursing, medical, nutrition, psychology and dentistry students and residents.

Research participants

Six parents of children admitted to the aforementioned paediatric unit took part in the study, meeting the pre-established inclusion criteria. In order to preserve the identity of the subjects, anonymity was guaranteed and all the participants were identified by fictitious names corresponding to children's characters.

Criteria for selecting participants

The participants in the research were those who met the following criteria:

- Have a child admitted to the paediatric unit at the time of the study;
- Have a child between the ages of 5 and 10;
  Having a child who is conscious, speaking and situated in time and space;
- Have a child who is not in isolation;
- Have agreed to take part in the proposed activities and have full and complete agreement to the child's participation in the study by signing an informed consent form;
- Agree to the presentation and dissemination of the results in academic and scientific circles.

Data collection procedure

Firstly, in order to carry out the study, the request form for research at the hospital was filled in online. After confirmation, authorisation to carry out the research was requested from the institution's head of nursing (Appendix A) and the education service (Appendix B) through a formal document setting out the purpose of the project.

With the institution's authorisation, a letter (Appendix C) was sent to the afternoon nurse at the unit in question to present the objectives of the study and ask for her permission to carry out the collection. Secondly, the project was sent to a Research Ethics Committee (Appendix D) and approved under opinion number 083/2012 (Appendix 1). After these assessments and the research being authorised, data collection took place.

Before collecting data from parents and hospitalised children, the author carried out play activities during the child's stay in the paediatric unit. The first approach was made during admission, using puppets and toys, and the child was invited to get to know the unit and the recreation room. This made the initial contact and the first procedures of anamnesis and physical examination easier for both the nursing team and the child. A playful approach was applied throughout the hospitalisation period, where they were encouraged to use their imagination and create a happier, less hostile reality. Using superhero masks, they created brave and strong characters, which helped during painful procedures. When procedures were necessary, the children went through a moment of preparation, explaining through games the objective and how the technique would be carried out.

By playing with hospital instruments and dolls, the children were able to experience and repeat the procedure by playing with the dolls or doing it to themselves in a symbolic way. The aim was for the children to gain knowledge about the care they were undergoing and to see it in a less threatening way.When it came to venipuncture, it was necessary to explain to the children how it would be done using the therapeutic toy technique. After the procedure and fixing the venous access, drawings were made on the adhesive plaster, where each child had the opportunity to leave it in the way they liked best, bringing the unknown hospital environment closer to their childhood universe.In this way, all the procedures the child underwent were explained in an educational and childlike manner, making him feel confident in the team and understand the importance of this activity for his treatment and recovery.In addition, to express their feelings about the change that illness had brought to their lives, they drew pictures, talked and played games. They repeated in make-believe the events they had been facing and played hospital games, where the children were the doctors and nurses and their colleagues and the dolls were the patients, thus creating a new meaning for hospitalisation.The data collection procedure started with a drawing made by the child, in which he was asked to draw how he felt about the hospital environment and the nursing staff. Afterwards, the author presented the child's drawing to the parents, who interpreted it, describing how they thought their child was experiencing hospitalisation. The parents then answered a semi-structured interview with open questions (Appendix F).According to Minayo (2010), interviews are dialogues between two or more people, with the aim of producing information that is pertinent to the research in order to achieve the proposed objectives. Semi-structured interviews allow the interviewer to approach the topic through open-ended questions, giving them the ability to discuss the issue in question.The interview was carried out during the child's hospitalisation, in a private room, using a tape recorder. The objective of the study was presented, and those who agreed to take part in the study signed the free and informed consent form (Appendix E), making them aware of all the terms described therein. The informed consent form was reproduced in two copies, one of which was kept by the research subject and the other by the project author. The data will be kept by the author for five (05) years.

Ethical principles

In this study, ethical precepts were maintained, based on the Code of Ethics for Brazilian Nursing Professionals of 2007, chapter III (teaching, research and technical-scientific production), articles 89, 90 and 91, which deal with responsibilities and duties, and articles 94 and 98, referring to prohibitions, and also in accordance with Resolution No. 196/96 of the National Health Council of the Ministry of Health, referring to research involving human beings.

Analysing the data

Data analysis was carried out with the aim of analysing the material collected, offering the researcher the possibility of investigating, broadening and deepening their understanding of the subject being researched, where they will be able to relate it to the cultural context of each person (MINAYO, 2010). According to the author, data analysis consists of three stages.

1st stage - Sorting the data: after obtaining the data, the content of the interviews will be read and explored, focusing on the objectives of the study. 2nd stage - Classification: coding and categorisation of the data by theme and through a theoretical basis. 3rd stage - Final analysis and interpretation: interpretation of the data using the literature review and the author's reflections.

CHAPTER 5 PRESENTATION, ANALYSIS AND DISCUSSION OF RESULTS

This section will present the discussion and analysis of the qualitative data obtained during the research, as well as the theoretical review of the subject. Firstly, the subjects participating in the research will be presented and then the following themes established after reading the material will be discussed: Playfulness **as a facilitator during hospitalisation in childhood, Playfulness as an auxiliary tool in treatment and prognosis, Playfulness as a working tool for nurses.**

Presentation of the Subjects

Mum/Dad	Minnie	Rapunzel	Tinkerbell	Monica	Robin	Fiona
Sex	Female	Female	Female	Female	Male	Female
Age	27 years old	28 years old	32 years old	34 years old	40 years	24 years old
Education	Teaching High School Completed	Teaching Medium Incomplete	Secondary school incomplete	High school incomplete	Incomplete primary education	Secondary school incomplete
Marital status	Single	Single	Single	Married	Widowed	Single
Occupation	Housewife	Owner of Home	Sales assistant	Hairdresser	Vigilante	Diarist
No. of children	02	01	04	02	03	02
Son hospitalised	Mickey	Cinderella	Peter Pan	Chives	Batman	Shrek
Sex	Male	Female	Male	Male	Male	Male
Age	08	07	10	09	10	05
Diagnosis	Haemophilia	Colitis Ulcerative	Crisis Asthmatic	Asthmatic Crisis	Leukaemia	Pneumonia
N° of hospitalisations	10	01	20	01	01	02

The study involved six (06) carers of children hospitalised in the Paediatric Inpatient Unit, the majority of whom were female (83%), aged between

24 and 40, most of whom had completed secondary school and were single (66%), with different professions, two of whom (33%) were housewives, with between one and four children. The majority of the children hospitalised were male (83%), aged between 5 and 10 years, with various diagnoses, 03 (50%) of which were for respiratory problems, with between 1 and 20 hospitalisations.

Play as a facilitator of hospitalisation in childhood

According to Motta and Enumo (2004), hospitalisation in childhood can interfere with quality of life and affect the child's healthy development. The child may face difficulties in their social and family life, as there are restrictions on socialising with other people, absences from school and increased distress and family tension. Added to this is the fact that they have to adapt to new schedules and routines, put their trust in previously unknown people, undergo invasive and painful procedures, as well as remain in a room where they are deprived of activities and see other children experiencing the same situation as them.

These feelings are expressed in the following statements:

> "Well... until a while ago it was very difficult to come to hospital [...] he wouldn't accept it, he was scared of everything." (Minnie, Mickey's mum)

> "Oh, it's hard for him because he's afraid of the medication and he also misses his family." (Mônica, Cebolinha's mother)

> "At first he was terrified [...] He was moved to see the babies here, with the same thing as him, with venous access in their arms. He'd never seen people like this, dressed in white. So everything is new to him." (Robin, Batman's father)

These statements are confirmed by Frota et al. (2007) when they say that hospitalisation is an unpleasant experience for the child, as they watch everything without having the power to make decisions or take initiatives, adding to the experience of hospital confinement, bringing up feelings of impotence, anguish and fear.

According to the author, one of the ways of helping children to clarify and cope with the changes they have experienced is through the use of play, with the aim of relieving fears and anxieties. It emerges as an attempt to transform the hospital environment through symbolic activity. Motta and Enumo (2004) report that playful components are stimuli for the child's positive adaptation to the hospital environment.

The benefits of play for children's adaptation to the paediatric inpatient unit are confirmed in the speeches:

> "He's reacted well now, he's fine [...] I even think he found the hospital quite lively because he drew the ball pool, the recreation room." (Minnie, Mickey's mum)

> "She's taking it well, she's finding it good, she's not depressed [...] she's identified well with the environment, especially the playroom." (Rapunzel, Cinderella's mum)

> "He's been feeling like this, he feels like he's at home [...] in the drawing he showed that he likes it here, especially this hospital. He likes it and says it's the best because of the recreation." (Tink, Peter Pan's mum)

> "He's become more cheerful and tells you that he 'feels' good, that he 'feels' at home" (Robin, Batman's father)

I therefore refer to Mitre and Gomes (2004) when they say that the act of playing is a way of transforming the reality and daily life of hospitalisation, since it reflects the unique reality of each child who shares a culture of play formed from the social environment in which they live.

By expressing themselves playfully, children relieve tension and stress, and according to Figueiredo (2010), play gives children the opportunity to express their emotions, show their needs, fears and desires. They are able to modify their thinking, taking the focus off illness and its consequences. According to Monica, Rapunzel and Fiona, while they were playing their children were no longer thinking only about the negative consequences of hospitalisation, because according to Mitre and Gomes (2004) play can be seen as a possibility to build something good at a time of so much loss:

> "Using the toys distracts him and he thinks about other things. It relieved the tension of being in hospital[...] He doesn't just think about his medication, he has other things to do. He goes to the toy room and

plays." (Mônica, Cebolinha's mum)

"Even with the pain she's being distracted and it's been very good for her [...] the games distract the children and she forgets about the pain." (Rapunzel, mother of Cinderella) (Rapunzel, Cinderella's mum) "He just stayed in bed and whimpered, wanting to go away. Now that he's started playing he doesn't talk about it all the time, he just asks to go to the playground and play." (Fiona, Shrek's mum)

In this sense, Frota et al. (2007) believe that play makes a contribution to minimising the trauma of illness and hospitalisation, offering children the chance to develop and grow healthily. Since playfulness is an alternative for resolving the conflicts encountered, it can be said that when children play, they are able to express their feelings and fears, feeling relaxed and happy, making their stay in hospital easier.

According to the following statements, it can be understood that the use of toys in the hospital environment played a fundamental role in providing distraction and entertainment for the children:

"With the toys, everything is a party for him [...] he showed in his drawing that he feels a bit more at ease in the play area." (Fiona, Shrek's mum)

"The use of toys distracts the children a lot, because they're no longer here because they want to be, they're already upset, they've got something (illness), they've got nothing to do. So the toys keep them very entertained." (Minnie, Mickey's mum)

"It's very good for her to play here because at least the games distract the children. She's not just stuck on the bed, she's distracted. Even if she's in pain, she goes and plays with other children" (Rapunzel, Cinderella's mum).

"The toys entertain the children, they have something to do. It gets boring sitting on the bed with nothing to do, they're stuck in their room. So here they go out, play for a while and play with each other." (Tinker Bell, Peter Pan's mum)

Tinker's view is also shared by Mitre and Gomes (2004) when they say that play functions as a space for socialising and interacting with other children, allowing them to create a new network of social relationships, creating the possibility of breaking out of the isolation caused by hospitalisation.

With regard to the well-being provided by the use of games, we can analyse Robin's speech:

> "The games are very distracting [...] my son even smiles now. He was sad and now you can see that he's always laughing, he's already excited about drawing [...] these are things that I think have to continue because they really help the children in hospital." (Robin, Batman's father)

This is in line with Mitre and Gomes (2004), who say that play is something pleasurable for children, brings joy and also rescues their own condition of "being a child". Playfulness becomes a counterpoint to the painful experiences of hospitalisation, which in this sense goes beyond the physical pain caused by the illness or the procedures to a concept of psychological and existential suffering.

According to Silva et al (2006), children's needs during hospitalisation remain the same as when they were at home, with a few more added as a result of hospitalisation or new situations that generate stress. At such times, play becomes essential in the child's development process, enabling them to restore and maintain their physical and mental health, keeping them active and exploring the new reality that surrounds them. In this context, it is essential to reflect that the act of playing brings benefits and makes the stay in hospital less hostile, providing pleasant feelings of fun as well as the opportunity to vent their anxieties, fears and insecurities.

Playfulness as an auxiliary tool in treatment and prognosis

In addition to the benefits for the child's adaptation to the Paediatric Inpatient Unit, play provides a pleasurable moment with a therapeutic function. According to Mitre and Gomes (2004), the act of playing is seen as therapy insofar as it is a way for children to elaborate on the experience of hospitalisation, allowing them to reorganise their feelings. It is an instrument capable of reassuring the child and making them lose their fear of the hospital. In addition, play is an action on the body itself, promoting a psychosomatic balance and helping to regulate tension and stress, having a direct effect on the immune system.

According to the following statements, we can see that, for the parents, play activities had a direct impact on their children's clinical condition:

> "The recreation room, getting the toys, drawing [...] I was surprised, if the recovery is 20 days, in less he can recover, the toys 'are' helping him a lot...a lot." (Robin, Batman's father) "I think it's good...for them it's good, right?...because he feels a bit better, a bit more at ease, because it helps too, as he goes there (recreation) it improves his health too." (Fiona, Shrek's mum)

According to Frota et. al (2007), the use of play promotes the child's overall development because it involves actions such as role-playing and allows the child to express what they are experiencing, thus having a healing function, acting as a means of escape and leading to a reduction in anxiety through emotional catharsis.

For Silva et al (2006), whatever the game, all the body's senses are stimulated, triggering emotions of euphoria, joy and well-being. Depending on these emotions, the body releases substances that are good for your health.

Therefore, play can improve the quality of life of these children, directly affecting their treatment. This statement is shared in the speeches below:

> "If you have an environment that makes you feel good and you can distract yourself with other things, the treatment is better." (Minnie, Mickey's mum)

> "He has to feel good spiritually too... then he feels more like it, he has more strength to heal himself... to get better... He feels a bit better, because before he went there (recreation room) [...] he was sad, he only had a fever, he just lay there. After he saw that there was a recreation room, he started to want to get up, go there, play, he started to walk more, he got better." (Fiona, Shrek's mum)

From Fiona's words, it can be seen that her son started to do more physical activity, became more willing, and started to feel more energised and better. On this point, Motta and Enumo (2004) state that from this child's point of view, the act of playing begins mainly because of the immediate effect of fun and entertainment it has on them. By playing, the child alters their environment and brings it closer to their everyday reality, having a very beneficial effect on their hospitalisation. As a result, the playful, free and disinterested activity itself takes on a therapeutic character, helping to promote the child's well-being.

On the other hand, for the authors, play can have a technical and therapeutic application, referring to its use with hospitalised children to help them understand and adapt more adequately to the invasive procedure. In this way, the toy is intended to introduce the procedure, explain its importance and provide opportunities for the child to ask questions and interact collaboratively during the technique. The benefits of using toys during painful procedures are expressed in Robin and Fiona's statements:

> "Doing activities, playing with him...making him laugh [...] he was stuck and now he's not...he's relaxed, he's happy to do the procedures." (Robin, Batman's father)

> "Playing makes it easier for you to examine him, right, and to treat him too... he gets better more quickly." (Fiona, Shrek's mum)

Based on the relevance of therapeutic play during procedures, Figueiredo (2010) assures that it is a way of connecting the scientific rationality of health practices with the subjectivity contained within each person, allowing treatment to go beyond technical procedures. The materials that commonly cause fear become toys, enabling children to face painful and invasive actions with the idea that it is also a game. Sharing this point of view, Mitre and Gomes (2004) say that play provides children with a language that is their domain, allowing them to make choices and become active agents in their own treatment. Therefore, the concern is not just to decorate the hospital environment, but to give children the chance to learn about and demystify procedures by participating interactively in play.

According to Frota et al. (2007), children face many difficulties during the period of illness, including painful and unpleasant experiences. These experiences make them feel helpless and in their imaginary childhood universe they take on threatening proportions. They often feel fragile and defenceless, prostrate and with their thoughts fixed on the illness.

In the words of the parents of hospitalised children, play can be found as a distraction mechanism, taking the focus off the illness and the treatment, and the child was able to achieve improvements in their health:

> "If he stays in bed, he'll think he's really ill. Playing gives him a bit of a break from that... there are children who get it into their heads that they have an illness and then it never heals... not with toys... it gives him a bit of a break, it takes his mind off it... that he's ill" (Tinkerbell, Peter Pan's mother).
>
> "The toy certainly helps with the treatment [...] It makes them feel better. The other little boy, for example, was sad and you brought him the toy jeep and he kept playing...so they forget about it (the illness) because in their little heads they think it's suddenly such a...serious thing, I know it's serious, but I don't know what's going on in their heads that they suddenly think they're going to die...thinking it's worse." (Robin, Batman's father)

In this way, Borges et al. (2008) share that play is capable of significantly reducing aggression, anguish and pain, which are characterised as losses resulting from hospitalisation, manifested through fear of the healthcare team, crying, aggression, dependence, pain, anxiety and sleep disturbances. In this scenario, play becomes fundamental as it guarantees joy and positively favours development and treatment, where play comes to be seen as a therapeutic space, capable of promoting the continuity of child development and giving the child the chance to get to know and adapt to the new environment, making a significant contribution to treatment and prognosis.

Play as a working tool for nurses

According to Castro and Almeida (2006), the nursing team has the privilege of being directly with the patient, having direct and continuous contact, implying a closeness that allows for equity and comprehensive care based on the principles of the SUS. To this end, it uses promotion, prevention and treatment to defend the health of paediatric clients. Bringing nurses and children closer together requires more than just technical components; it requires a different look and behavioural changes in relation to the little patient. In this scenario, it is essential to revive humanised care by confronting it with the technical and scientific development of today's society, which leads to fragmented tasks that lose sight of the individual.

According to the aforementioned authors, you can't allow adversity in your relationship with the child and avoid being a "cold", individualistic, calculating and biologicist professional. What is needed is professionals who have holistic care in mind, centred on the individual as a whole, with their unique and individual characteristics, which value the feelings and subjectivity of the human being, with the valuing of affectivity and sensitivity as the necessary elements of care.

Reinforcing the statements of the aforementioned authors, Góes and Cava (2009) believe that the care provided to hospitalised children needs to be based on a different model, centred on the child and their family, where actions should be comprehensive and not focus solely on the disease or the cure. It is of the utmost importance to look for personal and social factors that directly affect the child's health-disease process. To this end, nurses must maintain a relationship of dialogue and trust in order to provide quality care based on the real needs of the child and their family.

The importance of the bond, dialogue and the relationship of trust and friendship between child and nurse is expressed in Robin and Minnie's speech:

> "At home he was totally down and the moment he came in here, he saw happy people talking to him and looking after him [...] all the time...doing activities, playing games, messing with him...making him laugh, always lifting his spirits[....] he started to wake up, because he arrived here shy and afraid and then, you kept talking to him, saying 'my big friend', doing those greetings that they like...those little touches on the hand, those things, he started to loosen up." (Robin, Batman's father)

> "I thought it was really nice because on the first day he came straight in playing, he took him to the playground, he made friends with another little girl, they played games, things that if he hadn't he'd be isolated in his room, you know, on his own." (Minnie, Mickey's mum)

These actions developed by nurses should aim to humanise the service provided, where Castro and Almeida (2006) believe they should presuppose the development of essential human characteristics such as sensitivity, respect and solidarity with their fellow human beings in all aspects of human life. The development of solidarity and commitment to children implies a transformation in the way they are viewed, where they are seen as subjects with individualised needs that need to be met. A broader view of children's needs facilitates communication and makes it more effective between adults and children. Furthermore, this process of humanisation becomes essential during a time of hospitalisation, which leads to fragility and vulnerability.

According to Frota et al (2007), in an attempt to achieve humanisation in the care of hospitalised children, nurses have tools at their disposal capable of providing experiences with new objectives and sensations, using non-threatening activities and feelings. Playfulness brings the dynamics of interactions and is used as a means of articulating the child's treatment and cure. For Mitre and Gomes (2004), it is essential to promote play during nursing practice, since dealing with children requires adapting their routines and using child-friendly language. Play is a facilitator for interaction between professionals, children and family members, as it is a universal expression of joy that ends up spreading to family members. In this informal atmosphere, it is possible to have a better exchange and the relationship becomes richer, and children and family members start to believe more in what the nurse is doing.

In this sense, play also brings benefits to family members, since when they see their children smiling and in a happier environment, they feel that they are being well looked after and are more at ease. This perception was pointed out in the speeches:

> "It's been marvellous for me, because she's out there playing, she's not stuck, sad on the bed in pain." (Rapunzel, Cinderella's mum)

> "I feel good, because we feel bad when the doctors and nurses treat the children badly... here they treat them well, they play and that's treating them well... they talk to them while playing... that's very good, especially for the children." (Tinker Bell, Peter Pan's mum)

> "He's doing very well... and I really thought the atmosphere was top notch, top notch!" (Robin, Batman's father)

In terms of the relationship between children and nurses, Mitre and Gomes (2004) emphasise the importance of the association between play and affection, where playfulness can create a space of affection and emotion. The professional comes to be seen as someone "good" who is there to give affection and care, and no longer as someone who will make the child feel pain and go through painful situations. As a result, play can be used as a significant tool to deal with issues such as: comprehensive care, adherence to treatment, the establishment of bonds that facilitate dialogue between professional, child and family, the maintenance of children's rights established by the ECA, and it can help children to give new meanings to illness and hospitalisation.

The change in the professional's behaviour, where they start to attend to the child's inherent needs, also generates a behavioural change in the child, as they start to feel safe and supported. The statements below show that professionals who use play as a working tool are more successful in their nursing practice:

> "To always examine by playing... I think that's good, otherwise he'll cry, he'll shout and then it's worse... he won't let you, and then it makes things difficult. And playing is easier." (Fiona, Shrek's mum)

> "The games help him a lot when it comes to doing things, the procedures." (Tinker Bell, Peter Pan's mum)

> "She did a lot of things with you there (recreation). With the toys, the paintings, the dolls before the procedures...the ball pool, everything helps her a lot." (Rapunzel, Cinderella's mum)

> "Doing activities, playing games, messing with him... making him laugh [...] he's relaxed, he's happy to carry out the procedures." (Robin, Batman's father)

With this in mind, Frota et al (2007) point out that the professional-play-child triad is capable of interconnecting purposes and expectations, facilitating positive interaction, where play is the primary tool for humanised intervention, as it promotes a relationship between the real world and the imaginary world capable of overcoming the barriers of illness and hospitalisation. Viana, Leão and Figueiredo (2010) state that the use of play must be adapted to reduce the anxiety generated by hospitalisation and requires more than a recreational activity. It should be used by nurses who care for paediatric clients in accordance with the Resolution of the Federal Nursing Council (COFen) No. 295/2004.

The importance of the bond, feelings of friendship, trust and affection were expressed in the drawings made by the children, who received special attention with a playful approach:

"He had a playroom and you were always there helping him." (Minnie, Mickey's mum)

> "She did everything in the playroom, she made people, including you, right?" (Rapunzel, Cinderella's mum)

"In the drawing he tried to draw a nurse...that's you, right" (Mônica, Cebolinha's mum)

"He [...] made you here... he referred to you here... and the recreation room. You and the recreation room helped him a lot. Because 'like this'...even at school he's like this...he doesn't feel like writing, drawing...and here he drew a lot, you know? He doesn't usually have much interest and here he surprised me by showing an interest in doing this drawing that I asked him to do." (Robin, Batman's father)

As a result, it can be seen that the playful approach brought benefits to the children, as they showed how important this experience was during their hospitalisation, transforming a moment of fragility into joy and optimism.

Thus, Mitre and Gomes (2004) state that the choice of play as a working tool is directly linked to the nurse's concept of the human being. Thus, Frota et al (2007) point out that it is necessary to be involved throughout the therapeutic process, minimising the anguish of children and their families, with the children's universe as a priority.

It is therefore necessary to change the way we view childcare, taking into account the child's uniqueness and the way they experience illness and treatment. We need to look for new ways of caring, going beyond the barriers of the technical-scientific model and adding love, affection and companionship to the child's experience.

CHAPTER 6 FINAL CONSIDERATIONS

Hospitalisation is an episode surrounded by countless difficulties, and it gets worse when it occurs during childhood. Children's worlds are made up of fantasies, dreams and imagination, and in this sense, play becomes a fundamental part of a child's healthy growth and development. During hospitalisation, children's imaginations take on new proportions, where they begin to see the hospital in an individual and unique way, which can generate negative feelings and trauma.

This is why we realised that there was an inherent need for professionals to bring playfulness and all the necessary sensitivity to the cold and unknown universe of the hospital, bringing it closer to the world of children. Play has become a fundamental part of nursing care, capable of providing strong bonds, better adaptation, reducing anxiety, fear, aggression and sadness.

In addition, with the use of games, the nurse was seen as a friend who was there to help, making the child feel supported. Seen in this way, there was better acceptance of painful procedures, making the moment less impactful for the child. As well as trusting the professional, the child was guided through everything that would happen, feeling important and able to have a say in their treatment.

However, in relation to the objective of investigating the use of playful activities by the nursing team, it was realised that there are still difficulties in implementing play as a routine. As it is a new idea, professionals are reluctant to adopt it, leaving this task to the recreationalist alone. This attitude is the result of a biologicist view, where the child is seen as a sick patient who needs clinical care. Often, nurses are also overworked, which creates barriers for them to implement play activities in their work routine. What's more, during the investigation we realised that the entire perception reported by the parents was anchored in the activities carried out by the author during the hospitalisation of the children in this study. This led to the need to add the play activities carried out by the author to the methodology, since these influenced the parents' responses.

We believe that the aim of this work was achieved, since in their reports, the parents of the hospitalised children expressed the importance that the play activities brought during their child's stay in the paediatric unit. They report that the activities provided moments of fun, that their children became more animated, smiling and playing, and that they were able to recover the very condition of "being a child". As a result, the hospital environment became less hostile and threatening, facilitating the child's experience and their adherence to treatment.

The importance of the bond of friendship between the nurse, who proposes a playful approach, and the child was mentioned in the interviews, in which the parents expressed their gratitude for the way their children were treated during hospitalisation. For them, the relationship of trust and affection was fundamental for the best quality of care provided, positively favouring their children's quality of life.

By finalising this work, we had the opportunity to experience what children go through and how much they can suffer when they are not properly handled. Throughout their lives, nurses must take on board the real meaning of the word "care", focusing on the human being as a whole, with the basic principle of humanising their care. With regard to paediatric nursing, it is of the utmost importance to bear in mind that humanising means meeting all children's needs, where play is essential and indispensable so that the experiences of hospitalisation can be lived with all the magic of a child's universe of play and with smiles of joy.

REFERENCES

BOFF, Leonardo. **Knowing how to care** - ethics of the human - compassion for the earth. 17th Ed. Rio de Janeiro: Vozes, 2011. 200p.

BORGES, Emnielle Pinto et al. Benefits of playful activities in the treatment of children with cancer. **Bol. Academia paulista de psicologia.** V.28. n.2. São Paulo. December 2008.

BRAZIL, **Management and Managers of Public Policies for Child Health Care:** 70 years of history. 1st Edition. Brasília- DF, 2011.

BRAZIL, **State of the World's Children 2008: Brazil** Notebook. Brazil- DF, January

BRAZIL. **Statute of the child and adolescent:** Law n. 8.069, of 13 July 1990, Law n. 8.242, of 12 October 1991. - 3rd ed. - Brasília : Chamber of Deputies, Publications Coordination, 2001.

BRAZIL. Ministry of Health. **O SUS de A a Z Garantindo Saúde nos Municipios.** 3rd Edition. Brasília- DF, 2009.

BRAZIL. Ministry of Health. **National Health Care Secretariat. ABC do SUS -** Doctrines and principles. Brasília: 1990.

BRAZIL. Federal Senate. **Constitution of the Federative Republic of Brazil.** Text Promulgated on 5th October 1988. Brasília, 2010.

CANDEIAS,Nelly Martins Ferreira. Concepts of education and health promotion: Individual changes and organisational changes. **Rev. Saúde Pública.** v. 31 n. 2. São Paulo, Apr. 1997.

CASTRO, Amparito Del Rocio and ALMEIDA, Ana Paula. Use of Therapeutic Toys in Nursing Care for Clients. In: SILVA, Ana Paula et. al. . **Instituto da Criança 30 anos: Ações atuais na** Atenção Interdisciplinar em Pediatria. São Paulo: Yendis, 2006. 270p.

Code of Ethics for Nursing Professionals. COFEN Resolution No. 311/2007.

COLLET, Neusa. and ROCHA, Semiramis Melani. Hospitalised child: mother and nurse sharing care. **Rev. Latino- AM. Enfermagem.** 2004; 12(2):191-7.

FEDERAL NURSING COUNCIL. Provides for the use of therapeutic toys by nurses in the care of hospitalised children.

CRESWELL, John. **Research design**: qualitative, quantitative and mixed methods. 3.ed. Porto Alegre: Artmed/Bookman, 2010.

FERRAZ, Fabiane. et. Al. Cuidar educando em enfermagem: passaporte para o aprender/ educar/ cuidar em saúde. **Rev. Bras Enferm.** 2005;58(5):607-10.

FIGUEIREDO, Nébia Maria Almeida. **Nursing Practices Series:** Teaching how to care for children. Rio de Janeiro: Yendis, 2010. 416p.

FRANCO, Sérgio. **Constructivism and education**. 9th Ed. Porto Alegre: Mediação, 2004.

FREIRE, Paulo. **Pedagogy of autonomy:** knowledge necessary for educational practice. 43°Ed. Rio de Janeiro: Paz e Terra, 2011. 144p.

FREIRE,Paulo. **Pedagogy of the oppressed.** 46th Ed. Rio de Janeiro: Paz e Terra. 2006. 214p.

FROTA, Mirna .et al. Play as a facilitating tool in the humanisation of care for hospitalised children. **Cogitare Enferm.** 2007, jan/mar; 12(1);69-75.

GÓES, Fernanda. and CAVA, Angela Maria. Nurses' conception of health education in the care of hospitalised children. **Rev. Eletr. Enf.** 2009; 11(4): 932-41. Available at < HTTP://www.fen.ufg.br/revista/v11/n4/v11n4a18.htm> accessed on 08 May 2012.

LEOPARDI, Maria Tereza. **Metodologia da pesquisa na Saúde**. 2 ed. Florianópolis: UFSC, 2002.

LUDIC. In:LAROUSSE ÁTICA: **Dicionário de língua Portuguesa-** Paris: Larousse/ São Paulo: Ática, 2001.

MELO, Luciana and VALLE, Elizabete. Hospital Toy Library. In: ALMEIDA, Fabiane and SABATÉS, Ana. **Paediatric Nursing**: children, adolescents and their families in hospital. Barueri- São Paulo- Manole, 2008. 448p.

MINAYO, Maria Cecília. **The challenge of knowledge**: qualitative research in health. 12.ed. São Paulo: Hucitec, 2010. 407p.

MITRE, Rosa Maria. and GOMES, Romeu. Promoting play in the context of children's hospitalisation as a health action. **Ciência e Saúde coletiva**. 9(1): 147154, 2004.

MITRE, Rosa Maria. **Playing for a living**: a study on the relationship between seriously ill and hospitalised children and play. Master's dissertation. Fernandes Figueira Institute, Fiocruz, Rio de Janeiro, 2000.

MOTTA, Alessandra. and ENUMO, Sônia. Playing in Hospital: A Strategy for Coping with Children's Hospitalisation. **Psicologia em estudo**, Maringá, v. 9, n. 1, p. 19-28, 2004.

OLIVEIRA, Sâmela and DIAS, Maria da Graça. Play and its Implications for Emotion Regulation Strategies in Hospitalised Children. **Psicologia: Reflexão e Crítica**, 16(1), pp. 1-13, 2003.

PAPALIA, Diane and OLDS, Sally. **Human Development**. 8ª ed.Porto Alegre:

Artmed. 2006. 928p.

PAPALIA, Diane and OLDS, Sally. **The World of the Child:** From Infancy to Adolescence. 11th Ed. São Paulo- McGraw-Hill: Artmed, 2009. 578p.

PIAJET, Jean. **The formation of the symbol in the child: imitation, play and dream, image and representation.** 4th Ed. São Paulo: LTC, 2010.

QUEIROZ, Maria Veraci. and JORGE, Maria Salete. Health education strategies and the quality of care and teaching in paediatrics: interaction, bonding and trust in the discourse of professionals. **Interface- Comunic, Saúde, Educ.,** v.9, n. 18, p. 117- 30, jan/jun 2006.

RAPPAPORT, Clara Regina. **Developmental psychology:** The pre-school age. Vol 3. 13th Ed. São Paulo: EPU, 2002.

RAVELLI, Ana Paula. and MOTTA,Maria da Graça. Play and child development: A focus on music and nursing care. **Rev. Bras. Enferm** ,2005, Sep-Oct; 58(5): 611-3.

Resolution no. 196, of 10 October 1996. National Health Council. Available at <http://www.upf.br/cep/download/anexo-a.pdf> accessed on 27 October 2012.

Resolution no. 295, of 24 October 2004. Provides for the use of the therapeutic toy technique by nurses in the care of hospitalised children. Rio de Janeiro. Available at < http://site.portalcofen.gov.br/node/4331 > accessed on 01 June 2012.

RIBEIRO, Circéia. ALMEIDA, Fabiane. BORBA, Regina. Children and play in hospital. In: ALMEIDA, Fabiane and SABATÉS, Ana. **Paediatric Nursing:** children, adolescents and their families in hospital. Barueri- São Paulo- Manole, 2008. 448p.

RIBEIRO, Circéia, BORBA, Regina. and MAIA, Edmara. The therapeutic toy in child care: The meaning for parents. **Rev. Soc. Bras. Nurs. Ped**. v.6, n. 2, p. 75-83 São Paulo, December 2006.

SABATÉS, Ana. Reactions of the child or adolescent and their family to illness and hospitalisation. In: ALMEIDA, Fabiane. e SABATÉS,Ana **Enfermagem Pediátrica:** a criança, o adolescente e sua família no hospital. Barueri- São Paulo- Manole, 2008. 448p.

SEBER, Maria da Glória. **Dialogue with children and the development of reasoning.** 1st ed. São Paulo: Scipionel, 1997. 246p.

SILVA, Ana Paula Alves. **Instituto da Criança 30 anos: Ações atuais na** Atenção Interdisciplinar em Pediatria. São Paulo: Yendis, 2006. 270p.

VIANA, Dirce Laplaca; LEÃO, Eliseth Ribeiro, FIGUEIREDO, Nébia Maria Almeida. **Specialisation in Nursing:** performance, intervention and nursing care. V.1. São Paulo- Yendis, 2010, 560p.

WALDOW, Vera Regina, LOPES,Marta and MEYER, Dagmar. **Ways of caring, ways of teaching:** nursing between school and professional practice. Porto Alegre: Artes Médicas, 1995. 203p.

ANNEXES

42

Annex 1: Drawing of Mickey, aged 08, diagnosed with haemophilia, 10 hospitalisations.

43

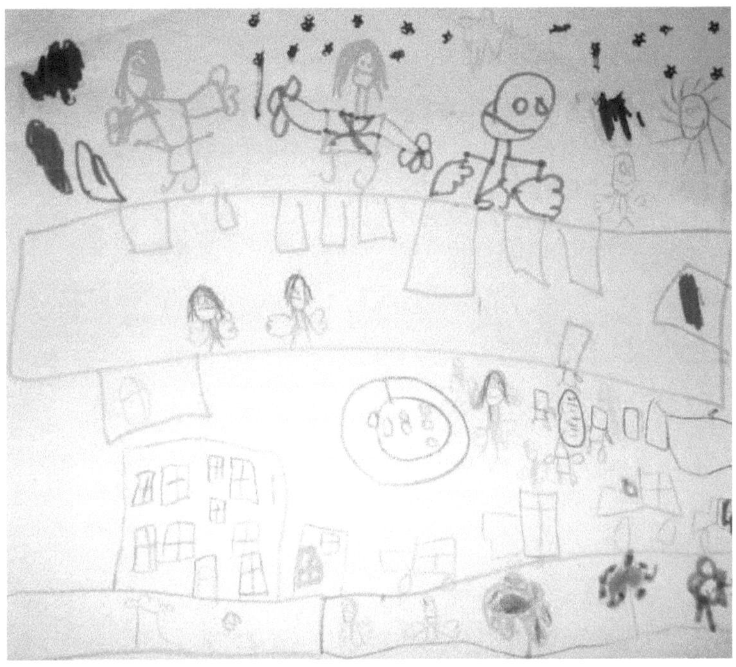

**Annex 2: Drawing of Cinderella, 07 years old, diagnosed with Ulcerative Colitis,
first hospitalisation**

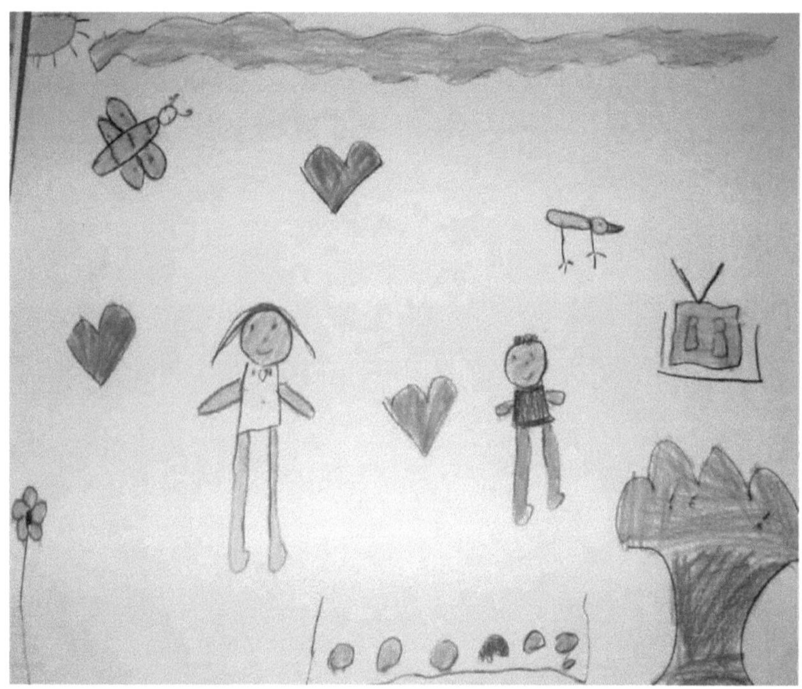

Annex 3: Drawing of Peter Pan, 09 years old, diagnosed with Asthmatic Crisis, 20 hospitalisations

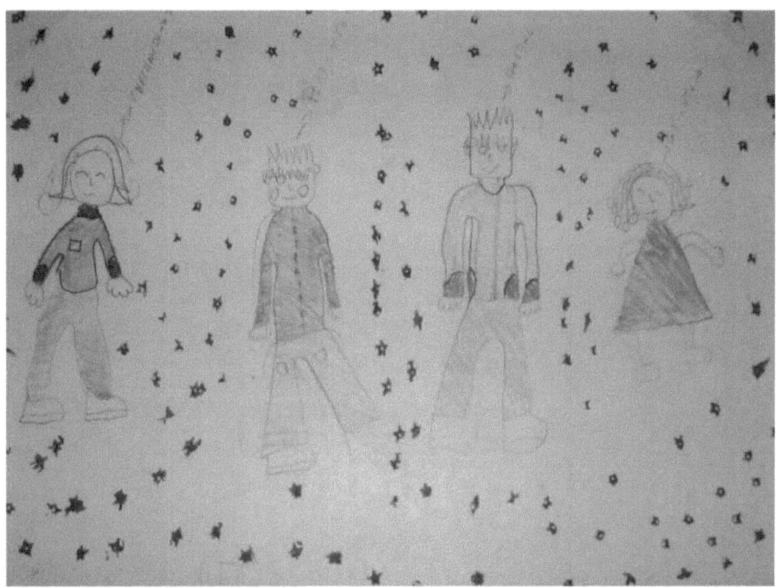

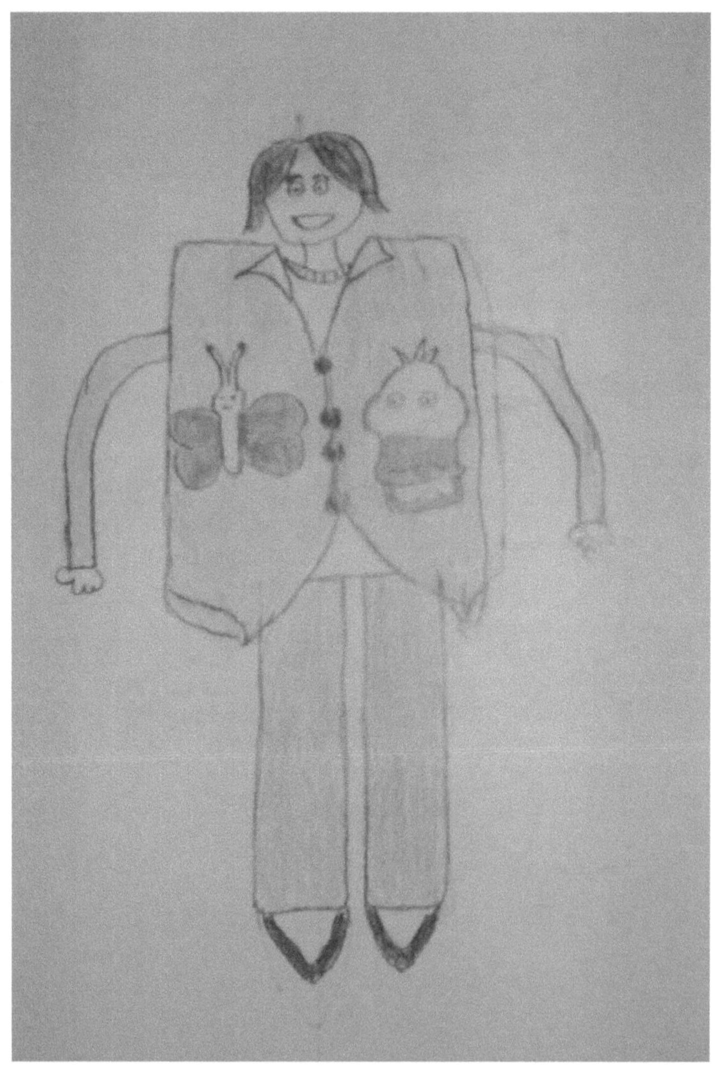

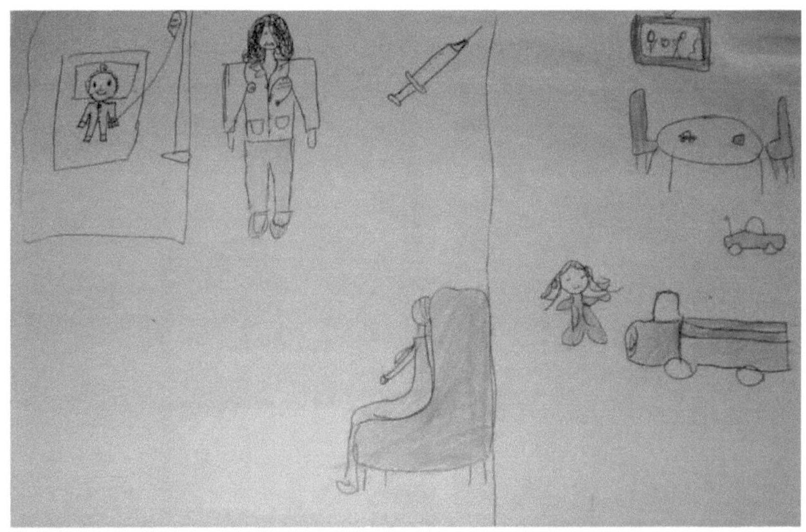

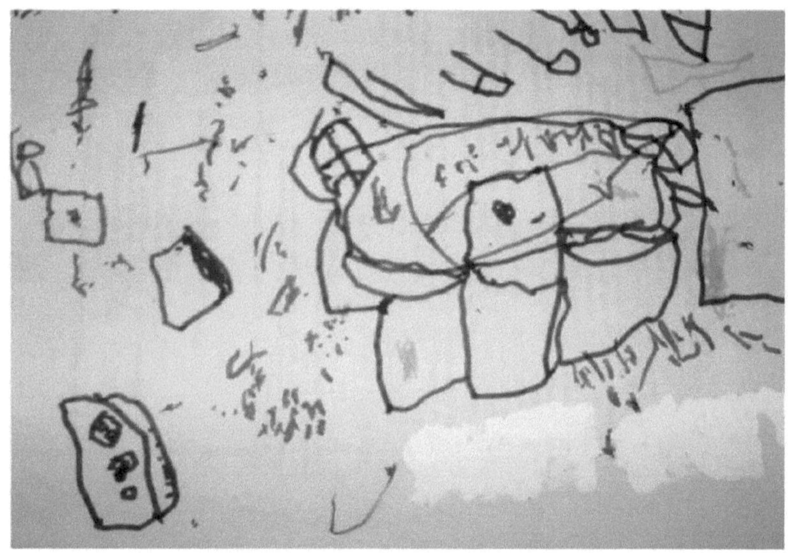

Table of contents

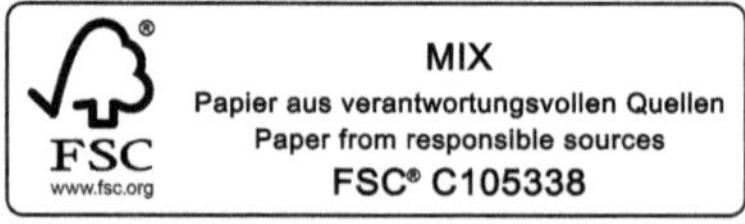

Printed by Books on Demand GmbH, Norderstedt / Germany